Yoga for Beginners

Beginners Essentials for Yoga

Dev Prisco

Warranty & Disclaimer

The author has made every attempt to be as accurate and complete as possible in the creation of this publication/PDF, however he/she does not warrant or represent at any time that the contents within are accurate due to the rapidly changing nature of the Internet AND the contents is for information value ONLY.

The author assumes no responsibility for errors, omissions, or contrary interpretation of the subject matter herein. Any perceived slights of specific persons, peoples, or organizations other published materials are unintentional.

This information is not intended for use as a source of MEDICAL, health fitness, legal, business, accounting or financial advice. All readers are advised to seek services of competent professionals in MEDICAL, health fitness, legal, business, accounting, and finance field.

No representation is made or implied that the reader will do as well from using the suggested techniques, strategies, methods, systems, or ideas; rather it is presented for news value only. The health aspects of Yoga are known but you MUST consult a medical doctor prior to beginning any exercise regimen including consulting an exercise physiologist, physical therapist and certified Yoga instructors for expert guidance.

Never attempt any health regimens, poses or ANYTHING based on ANY of the contents herein without first

consulting said mentioned experts in health, fitness and medical fields.

The author does not assume any responsibility or liability whatsoever for what you choose to do with this information. Use GOOD and consulted (expert) judgment.

Consult appropriate professionals before starting any exercise.

Any perceived remark, comment or use of organizations, people mentioned and any resemblance to characters living, dead or otherwise, real or fictitious, is for information value ONLY and used as examples only. There are no guarantees health benefits or promises of any kind. Readers are cautioned to reply on their own judgment about their individual circumstances to act accordingly and again are cautioned to include health professionals.

DISCLAIMER

Please note the information contained within this document is for educational purposes only. Every attempt has been made to provide accurate, up to date and reliable complete information no warranties of any kind are expressed or implied. Readers acknowledge that the author is not engaging in rendering MEDICAL, legal, financial or professional advice.

By reading any document, the reader agrees that under no circumstances is the author responsible for any losses, direct or indirect, that are incurred as a result of use of the information contained within this document, including - but not limited to errors, omissions, or inaccuracies.

Contents

Introduction

"Yoga is almost like music in a way; there's no end to it." –Sting

If you have been considering changing your life with Yoga, then this fantastic book will help you discover everything you need to know about the power of Yoga in your life.

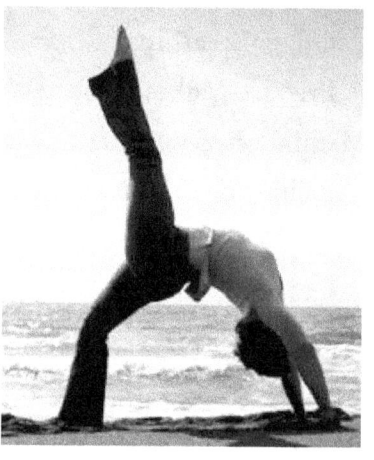

Yoga is not just about exercise but it encompasses inner peace, strength, meditation and spirit.

For many people who have not had enough flexibility or they feel constantly tired, Yoga is a way for them to change that aspect of themselves. It empowers us through movement, breath and energy focus.

For other people who have been practicing Yoga for a time and want a deeper connection to everything around them, the discipline is a way to understand a greater spiritual connection. Yoga is about transforming one's inner thoughts and bringing peace and tranquility to their lives through poses, breath and intention.

In this book we will go over some of the finer points of Yoga, give you an interesting explanation on the history and about Yoga's origins.

We would ask one thing of you; that you already visualize the transformation from day one of your physical and mental changes. Your first lesson with yoga is to know you are already a different person and you can achieve anything with the right commitment. Yoga is not just about the exercises but about the complete embodiment of what can happen to a person when they truly understand what it teaches. I would encourage you to think more positively on your thoughts, feelings and the ultimate connection to your inner power.

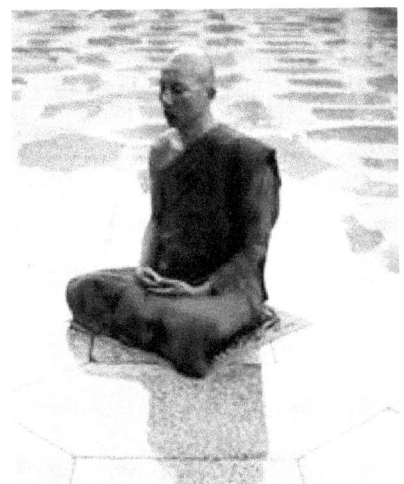

Posture and breathing is only part of what you will learn; but also you can discover real peace, focus and deeper meditation. For people who understand the meditation part of Yoga, they are naturally transformed because they will seek the deeper practices of enlightenment that the physical part provides to the mind.

If you do not believe that meditation is necessary to achieve higher levels in Yoga then you only need look at a Buddhist monk to see how meditation transforms their whole lives. Some of the Yogi's who achieve spiritual enlightenment can withstand pain, go many days without eating and drinking and can do physical things that many of us will never understand. It is a test of their will, knowledge and connection.

The Buddhist monks are some of the most disciplined and joyful people alive. They are giving and caring as well. They have inner peace because they experience the benefits of meditation and the special power harnessed from this connection.

Yoga is something families can enjoy together. Many children now are learning yoga poses because parents find the child can focus better by learning this type of discipline. This kind of peace can greatly improve a child's mental processing.

Yoga is an excellent practice for pregnant women. The poses definitely help in the birthing process and reduce pain in the lower back, while helping the hips to expand better. Yoga can reduce fatigue and help the expectant mother sleep better.

There has to be something important to yoga because for thousands of years many of the ancient cultures practice yoga. Whether it was from India, Egypt, Tibet or Burma, Yoga was practiced in unison as critical to daily living.

There is evidence that Yoga may be as old as 10,000 years. In this book we will touch on some of the history and why these ancient people connected to this most amazing way to live. Yoga is the ability to interconnect everything in our world and universe and soon you can too.

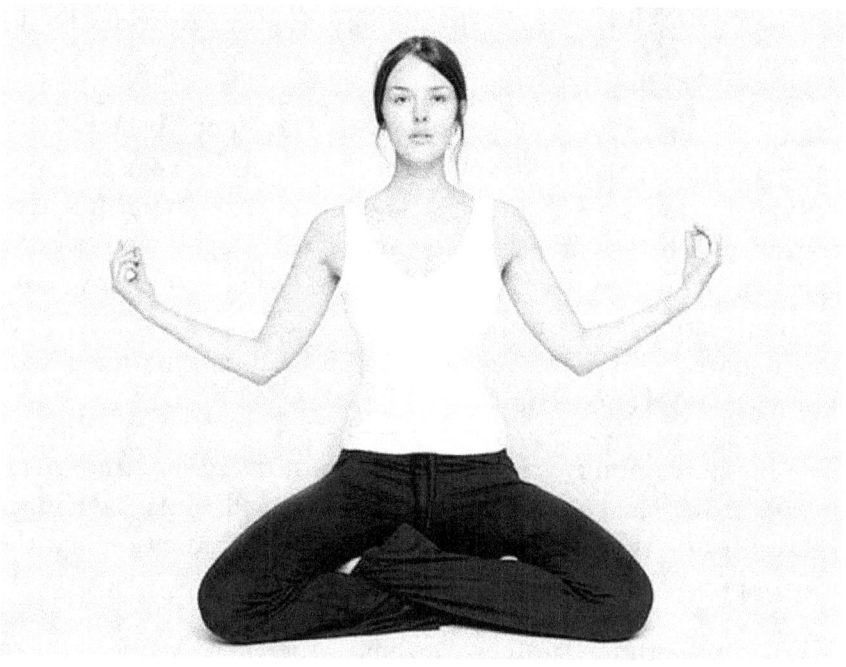

How Yoga Came To Be

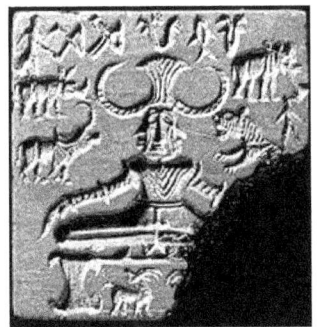

Millions of people around the world practice Yoga on a daily basis for better health, strengthening the body, connection, meditation and healing. The traditional purpose of Yoga has always been to bring about profound transformation in a person.

To think that Yoga is just about posture, poses and breathing is really not to know the real essence of it. Many people are surprised when they find that Yoga initiates a deeper connection to the inner spirit.

The actual word **Yoga** came from the East and it is reported that it was used by shaman over 3,000 years ago for all types of healing.

There have even been older seals found which are approximately dated around the mid-3rd millennium BCE which depict poses of a common meditation sitting position used in the discipline.

In Buddhism the word Yoga means "Spiritual Discipline." In Vedic Sanskrit, Yoga means "to add, to join, to unite or to attach."

Kemetic Yoga is reported to be as old as 10,000 years and was practiced by the Nubians and Egyptians. All thoughts and feelings were introduced through meditation which was practiced by the priestesses and priests. The people in this time actually referred to themselves as "Kemet" and the name Egyptian came later.

The Kemetic people believed that Yoga was the personal integration of oneself into the binding of the larger universal consciousness. In other words Yoga to these people was a system of discipline which transformed a person into the greater awareness to all that is. Kemetic Yoga's original intention is to lead a person into state of awakening which is called the "Nehast."

Human thought can change frequently if untrained and left to its own devices. A greater balance is needed to help the body through some the poses. One of these balances is the ability to sit, compose one's thoughts and meditate on healing and complete transformation.

Namaste is the Sanskrit word (over 4000 years old) used when the hands are clasped together in a prayer position near the heart chakra. Namaste means "Namah" means to bow or reverential salutation and "te" means to you. "I bow or salute you," or *The divine in me recognizes the divine in you.*"

Deciding on what style of Yoga to practice is a personal choice. Some people may feel comfortable with Hatha Yoga where others may need more invigoration for the body such as Bikram. Whatever decisions you make will become a part of your intention.

Large Yoga classes held in gyms and buildings are limited. The choice for the student to walk their own path is in part under what the teacher brings to the student. The personal connection through the meditation is not as intense because of the shared thoughts and energy within the room and less focus.

The benefits of these classes help the student to understand the poses better. For people who wish to become teachers themselves, larger classes offer the student the ability to learn correct posture and stance from the poses.

Doing Yoga practice alone is good for the meditational aspect. Remember that Yoga is about balance in all things. Alone time in Yoga is also strongly encouraged.

Health Benefits Of Yoga

Before anyone enters into a Yoga practice they should always first consult with their doctor to make sure they are healthy enough to begin. In rare cases Yoga should not be attempted for people who may have suffered from previous injuries or chronic strains to their back, neck and shoulders. Still, you should consider the needs of your body for healthy exercise. Yoga encompasses every kind of aspect your body needs to be healthy while allowing you to grow at your own pace. This is why many people love Yoga and practice it daily.

I recently became aware of Arthur Boorman a former disabled veteran because of his inspirational video on YouTube. Arthur was told he would never walk again without aid. He could only walk with knee braces and supports. He took this as a fact until he asked for help from a Yoga instructor . . . it forever changed his life.

We would like to share with you this video to prove to you what you can do and change your life when you believe in your own inner power:

www.youtu.be/qX9FSZJu448

Yes, Yoga can greatly improve the lives of almost anyone at any age or physical condition. You can expect to see any and all of these issues get better:

- High blood pressure

- Lower cholesterol levels

- Greatly reduce stress and depression

- To lose weight

- To have better skeletal alignment

- Improve strength and muscle tone

- To become more centered in everyday life

- Need better mental focus

- Spiritual connection through meditation

Yoga . . . A Powerful Ally To Your Health

There have been reported astounding health benefits from people who suffer from diabetes, cancer, muscle, skeletal problems and asthma by practicing Yoga.

A continual Yoga practice of a minimum of 3 times a week has greatly helped in the reduction of their diseases. Much of this research can be backed up from medical studies. Yoga is very, very good for you.

Yoga can also greatly improve the lives of people who suffer from depression and other types of mental illness because it brings calm and peace unlike any over the counter or prescription drug with no real side effects. Yoga also encourages daily meditation to help clarify ones thoughts and feelings, something few people take the time to do in our pressure cooker lives.

There have been numerous studies and research done on Yoga from the Departments of Psychology in the University of Connecticut, Samueli Institute, Alexandria, VA and Osher Institute at the Harvard Medical School. There are many other universities that have all concluded the benefits of Yoga on a person's health is without question – something few fad like exercises can totally say.

You can look at the PDF studies here:

www.sytar.org/syr2013/documents/SYR-Abstracts2011.pdf

Type 2 Diabetes A Killer To Millions

People who suffer from Type 2 Diabetes often have problems with nerve damage related to high sugar levels. Yoga has been found to stimulate and increase nerve impulses. The high sugar levels contribute to slower impulses, numbness in the feet and less sensations generally occurring in the body.

The Department of Physiology at the University College of Medical Sciences in Guru Tegh-Bahadur Hospital in Delhi, did research into Yoga and Type 2 diabetes. Five doctors were part of the research team who studied the effect of Yoga asanas on nerve conduction in diabetes.

These research studies were conducted in 2002, which proved that a regular Yoga regime for 40 days can improve nerve function and glycaemic index control in people suffering from mild type 2-diabetes. The test involved 20 people who were all type 2 and from the age of 30 to 60 years.

Every morning, for 40 days, patients would practice Yoga asanas for 30 to 40 minutes. The patients who practiced Yoga had improved results over those who practiced light exercise like walking.

Source: http://www.ncbi.nlm.nih.gov/pubmed/12613392

Oxidative Stress Is Reduced With Yoga

Oxidative stress causes free radicals to run wild in our body which can disrupt normal body functions, break down our cells and eventually lead to illnesses. This type of stress releases harmful chemicals which attack our bodies' immune systems, causes arthritis, heart problems and eventual saggy skin. We are also prone to more infections and eventual problems with our DNA from oxidative stress.

Building up a healthy immune system is essential in fighting oxidative stress disease and infection. Practicing Yoga on a regular basis can help the body fight free radicals through the poses.

These poses are designed to burn oxygen more slowly, encourage breathing techniques and reduce glucose loss as is the case with many other forms of exercise. Yoga actually helps the body to heal faster from the effects of stress and infection.

When meditation is added to the yoga practice it encourages a slowed metabolic rate. This greatly reduces free radicals and allows the body to eliminate them better through relaxed and deep breathing. Oxygen is slowly being released through your body from yoga while reducing your heart rate. The end result is better looking skin with a younger appearance, healthier body and greatly reducing free radicals.

Fibromyalgia Is Eased

If anyone suffers from Fibromyalgia then they are already aware of the total widespread musculoskeletal pain, tiredness, depression and anxiety associated with the disease. Fibromyalgia is one of those conditions that doctors are still learning about. An 8 week Hatha yoga study was carried out on women suffering with different levels of Fibromyalgia pain. Most of the women were also on prescribed pain medication. The results found that there was a significant reduction of the Cortisol hormone. Cortisol has been contributed to an increase in stress levels which then suppresses the immune system and causes more pain to the muscles.

Arthritis Is Lessened And Controlled

Yoga has the ability to lessen arthritis by creating more mobility within the joints. This increases a person's flexibility and strengthens the joints. It may also have the effect of lessoning the swelling that comes from arthritis and minimize some of the effects of erosion from the cartilage which causes the pain. Once upon a time people who suffered from joint pain were told not to exercise the muscles but that proved to be very bad advice. People who suffer from any form of joint or muscle pain must move and stretch the muscles in order to remain strong and healthy. When the muscles and joints are not used they actually become more painful. With regular Yoga poses and careful movement this encourages blood circulation and helps with better functioning of the immune system.

Breast and Ovarian Cancer Managed

Many women have claimed they were able to manage their pain better when they practiced Yoga after breast cancer surgery. Part of the healing process was for women to visualize all muscle and cells healed through the process of meditation. The breathing and slow intentional movements were also a part of the program. Restorative Yoga was the preferred choice for the healing aspects involved.

Here is a passage from the study: "Further, a recent pilot study of breast and prostate cancer patients who participated in mindfulness based stress reduction (relaxation, meditation, gentle yoga) demonstrated improvements in overall quality of life, symptoms of stress, and sleep quality."

With the increased availability of yoga programs for patients to practice; for the amount of research data in this area, yoga is essential healing in the process of cancer.

We found this excellent downloadable PDF named *"Restorative Yoga for Women with Ovarian or Breast Cancer: Findings from a Pilot Study;"* Please click on the link provided if you wish to read:

Source:
http://mahashakti.co.uk/wpcontent/uploads/2011/09/restorativ e_yoga_for_women_with_cancer.pdf

Patients with Lung Cancer

With the breathing techniques carried out in Yoga, studies have shown that patients who practiced this type of breathing did extremely well. The study was done on patients with a 45 minute workout with Hatha yoga. The shortness of breath eased and the breathing techniques applied through Hatha Yoga saturated the body with oxygen. Oxygen saturation remained high and vital signs stable and then increased significantly over the 14-week study period.

Depression Is Overcome Without Drugs

Yoga can be a positive way to beat depression. There are many people in this world who have suffered from depression and if not treated can be life threatening. Unfortunately many of the drugs used to treat depression have serious side effects. If you are a person who doesn't want to take medication for depression or other similar symptoms like anxiety, Yoga can help.

There are many Medical professionals who believe that depression can be related to a serotonin imbalance. Serotonin acts like a neurotransmitter that relays messages from one part of the body to the other. The theory is, if there is an imbalance it will affect mood, feelings and thoughts.

Princeton neuroscientist Barry Jacobs, PhD, says depression may occur when there is a suppression of new brain cells. Dr Jacobs also believes that stress is the most dominant culprit of depression.

Source:

www.psych.princeton.edu/psychology/research/jacobs/case.php

To relieve stress symptoms, practice yoga 3 to 4 times a week. This can greatly improve the health of anyone with depression. Yoga has been shown to help people who suffer from anxiety, Obsessive Compulsory Disorder (OCD) and other similar types of problems. By using the Ujjayi breathing technique, it can actually bring a sense of calm and peace to the body. It calms the stress response system way down. From studies done on women with psychiatric problems, once they practiced yoga regularly; these women showed significant improvement with depression and anxiety.

Source:

www.irest.us/sites/default/files/YogaNidra%20CAM%20anxiety_depres%20sm.pdf

Different Kinds Of Yoga

In a short time yoga can shape your body and give you a toned effect without all the straining and tearing muscle that weight lifting can do. Many of the Yoga poses use your own body weight as a way to increase your endurance and build muscle in a gentler, kinder way.

There are different types of yoga practices depending on breathing, spiritual consciousness and body movements you are trying to achieve. We are going to touch on some of the more popular types of yoga practice in this book. Depending on your goals, you too could become a Yoga Master Practitioner in time.

Ashtanga Yoga - Ashtanga got its name from the eight limbs of yoga, which were mentioned in the Yoga Sutras of Patanjali. It is a more modern form of classical Indian Yoga. You may have also heard the term "Power Yoga." Ashtanga is physically challenging to the body and many ex-athletes may prefer this type of yoga. The poses are based in a specific set of asana to move into a dynamic flow of movement. Some of these movements are also incorporated into Vinyasa Yoga.

Vinyasa Yoga - Most people will know the names "Vinyasa flow" these poses were brought to light by K. Pattabhi Jois and they quickly became popular poses. In Vinyasa people move gracefully from one pose to the other. Usually the classes are very different except for starting with sun salutations. Vinyasa is one of the most popular yoga practices and many teachers will use more of these poses in gyms and small centers.

Hatha Yoga – This form of Yoga incorporates slower and gentler movements. Mature people may prefer this type of Yoga because it is very calming on the body. Hatha yoga may also be a better choice for people to start out with, if they have had a previous medical injury. Hatha yoga is ideal to practice at night before sleep as it brings contentment and peace.

Bikram Yoga - If you like to sweat then Bikram is yoga designed to be practiced in 40% humidity and up to a 100 degree heat. There are only a total of 26 poses in Bikram but it concentrates more on the alignment work. There are facilities where it is not uncommon to see 50 or more people join the class doing Bikram yoga. Because it gets pretty hot inside the building don't be surprised if you see people working out in bikinis and swimwear.

Restorative Yoga - This type of Yoga helps the body calm down after a long day at work. Most of the principles are based in relaxation, peacefulness of mind and good breathing techniques. Medical studies have been carried out with recorded health benefits in treating cancers by practicing restorative yoga.

Prenatal Yoga - If you are expecting a baby, prenatal yoga is one of the best exercises you can do to prepare for birth. Most of this yoga concentrates on breathing and core exercises designed to prepare you for labor. Prenatal yoga can also help women with strength and flexibility, improve sleep patterns and decrease back pain. Many medical professionals now recommend Yoga as an excellent form of exercise for pregnancy and birth.

Kundalini Yoga - Is also referred as "Laya Yoga" from the Sanskrit name "dissolution and extinction." Many practitioners call it the yoga of awareness. Studies on Kundalini Yoga can help in treating psychiatric disorders. The intent is to raise individual awareness and embrace the potential strength in humans. It also raises the unconscious spiritual state in meditation.

We have previously mentioned **Kemetic Yoga** which incorporates a more spiritual universal connection into the poses along with daily consciousness within this ancient practice. In some ways Kundalini and Kemetic yoga are along the same spiritual pathways into healing mental disorders.

How Yoga Strengthens
Your Body Gently

Each pose in yoga is designed to help your body for strength, flexibility, focus and longevity. The breathing helps with the oxygen flow to the body and organs. It has been said there are over 1000 different recorded poses in yoga.

There are different asanas you can do that will work in specific ways for the body. Standing poses encourage the body to feel empowered for the day. Supine poses are known for their restorative powers. Core poses strengthen the abdomen and back. Twists help the body with strength and flexibility.

Many people like to take early morning yoga classes where the instructor will do a series of these types of poses. Each pose has a relationship to the other but what is more important is their relationship to you as you practice the poses.

You will never see a good teacher go from a standing pose to a hip opener in just 2 poses. You work a series of movements from each set of poses and then gradually move into the next set. We will give you an idea of what poses you can do in sequences.

You do not have to follow exactly what is here but rather these poses will show you where they belong within each set of asana's.

If you have already decided to start your own set of Asana's then we would suggest that you have a note book handy and write down the poses you believe you are capable of starting. Write down how you feel these poses will help you both physically and mentally. As your Yoga practice increases you may then add more intense poses as the body strengthens.

If you are committed to adding meditation into your yoga practice then decide how much time you will allow for this too.

Start with 5 to 10 minutes after you have completed the poses and gradually building up more time for a peaceful and tranquil state of mind.

We will name some of these poses in English and then place their Sanskrit names along side of them for you to learn. If you would like to see more poses and how to begin the positions I have provided a link to a site that will go through many of the poses from A to Z here: Poses Here

Even if you cannot do all the yoga poses on the floor to begin with, or you find it hard to cross your legs, do some of the sitting poses in a chair. This will still help with flexibility until the day comes when you can manage some of the floor poses.

Starting yoga in a chair can help people who have disabilities or problems with walking. Many senior citizens who have been bed ridden for quite some time can greatly benefit from starting yoga in a chair.

For pregnant women with back problems yoga can be done on an exercise ball. This takes the pressure off the spinal and pelvic areas of the body.

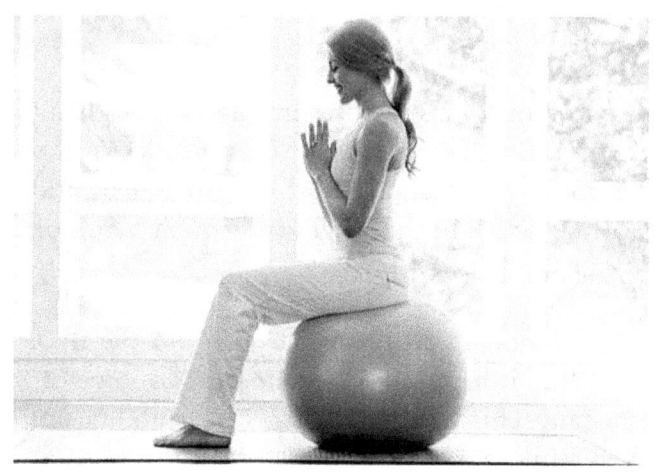

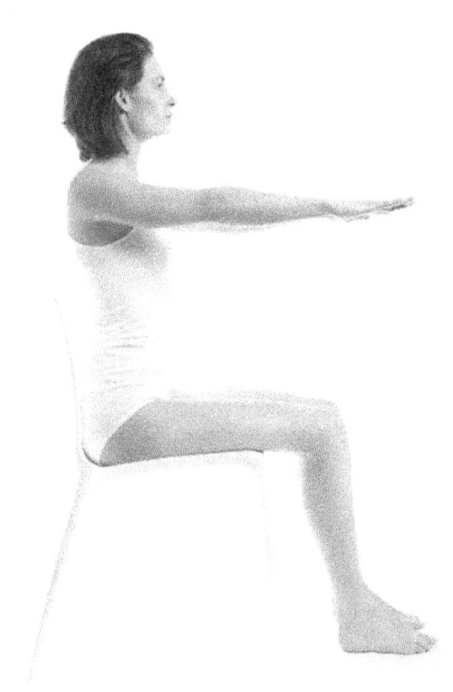

Standing Poses:

Triangle Pose (Trikonasana)

Warrior Pose I and II (Virabhadrasanas)

Tree Pose (Vrksasana)

Crescent Lunge Pose (Anjaneyasana)

Half   Moon   Pose   (Utthita Trikonasana)

Side Angle Pose (Parsvakonasana)

Sun Salutation (Surya Namaskar)

Chair Pose (Utkatasana)

Mountain Pose (Tadasana Samasthiti)

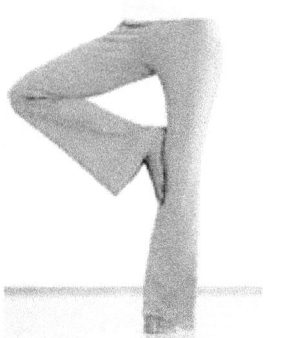

Standing poses are designed to be energetic poses

- Use large muscle groups.

- They help to provide a straight line of movement as we shape our bodies.

- These poses are also great for balance, strengthening muscles like arms, shoulders, thighs and legs.

- The poses also teach us the correct stance and focus.

The practice of the standing poses in yoga is an excellent way to help people develop more mobility from their joints. Standing poses help with the correct alignment of the spine. Positions like Warrior I and Warrior II encourage strength in the back, shoulders, arm muscles and legs. Warrior I, II and III poses also encourage the student to take on the persona of the spiritual warrior. Many times the student is mentally encouraged to visualize themselves as an ancient warrior in these poses.

People may find these poses difficult at first, especially if they tend to have shoulder pain. Do not expect more from yourself than is physically possible. Remember that Yoga is about bringing inner peace to your body and not straining in constant pain. We do not want you to think upon Yoga as a practice of pain but rather the total healing process of your body.

Seated Poses:

Boat Pose (Paripurna Navasana)

Staff Pose (Dandasana)

Hero Pose (Virasana)

Cobbler Pose (Baddha Konasana)

Easy Pose (Sukhasana)

Childs Pose (Balasana)

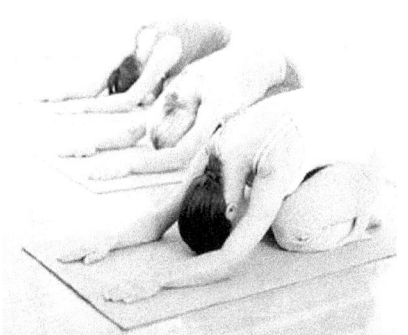

Seated   Forward   Bends
(Paschimothanasana)

Lotus Pose (Padmasana)

Garland Pose (Malasana)

Sitting Poses Can Benefit The Body In This Way:
- Flexibility and strengthen the spine
- Opening of the hips
- Massage the internal organs
- Help the body become more relaxed
- Seated poses can be used for meditation

Many seated poses in yoga are suitable for beginners. Seated yoga poses are based more in flexibility than strength. These poses tend to be more on grounding your body like a tree root is into the ground. The seated poses help a person to become more intent on focusing energy.

Many of the seated poses benefit the spine because you are required to keep it in straight alignment, which then stretches the muscles around the spine. These poses also help increase flexibility and reduce stress.

Body Twists:

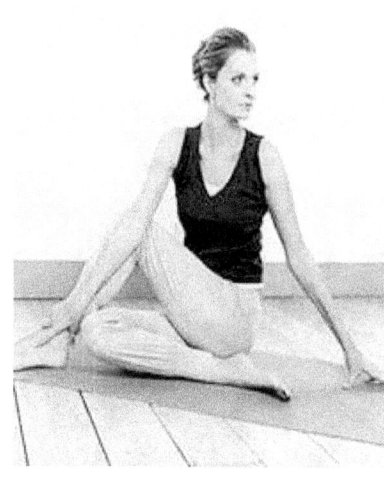

Half Twist Pose (Ardha Matsyendrasana)

TWISTED CHAIR POSE (Parivrtta Utkatasana)

Fish Pose (*MATSYASANA)*

LOCUST POSE (Poorna-Salabhasana)

Bow Pose (Urdhva Dhanurasana)

Eagle Pose (Garudasana)

The Benefits Of Twists:

- Increases flexibility in each vertebrae of the spine

- Twists stretch the back muscles and hips

- Strengthens the abdominal muscles, organs and relieves constipation

- Speeds up circulation as the breathing increases

- Brings more blood flow into the spine

- Increases metabolism and burns fat

- Soothes the nerves

(You should never end your practice with twists because they are usually related to the spine and your body requires a gentler way to relax. Many yoga poses will finish with relaxation or corpse pose.)

Many of the poses are spinal twists which can require supervision from a teacher.

If you are doing yoga in the home make sure that you have your feet securely positioned because these poses require you to remain grounded.

Breathing correctly before attempting your twist will allow you to move into position better. Keep breathing through the twist which will allow you to turn your body even more.

Supine Poses:

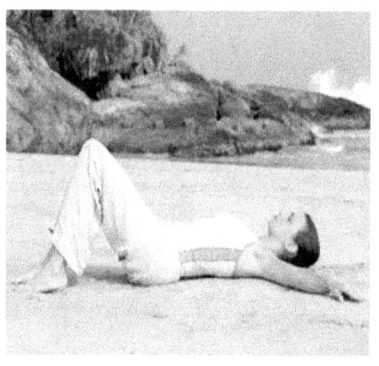

(MEANS LYING ON YOUR BACK POSES)

*BRIDGE POSE (*Setu Bandhasana)

Reclining Big Toe Pose (Supta Padangusthasana)

Legs Up The Wall Pose (Viparita Karani)

Plow Pose (Halasana)

Happy Baby Pose (Ananda Balasana)

Corpse Pose (Savasana)

Wind Relieving Pose (Pavanamuktasana)

The Benefits Of Supine Poses

- Develop *BODY* control

- Muscle tone, coordination

- Increases concentration levels

- Energizes the body

- Strengthen the arms, back and neck

- Stretches the abdomen and aids in mobility of the spine and hips

Single and double leg raises help prepare the body for asana's. They benefit the middle and lower back, legs and abdominal muscles. These poses will also support the hips and aid in spinal flexibility. The circulation in the body is also increased along with respiration.

The wind relieving pose will work on the digestive system and helps to rid the body of extra gas in the intestines.

The legs up the wall pose are entirely supported by the pelvic area and the hands, while the upper body is completely flat on the floor. This pose is ideal for pregnant women after they have passed the first trimester. Remember to place a pillow under your buttocks and forehead for better comfort.

Other Types Of Poses

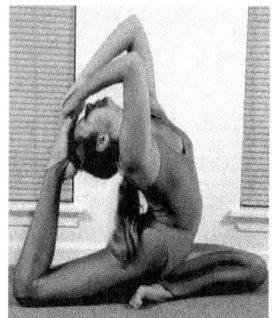

Standing Forward Bend (Uttanasana)

Seated Forward Bend (Paschimottanasana)

Wide-Legged Forward Bend (Prasarita)

Camel Pose (Ustrasana)

Upward Bow (Urdhva Dhanurasana)

Prone Poses (Lying on your stomach)

Forward Bend Benefits:

A forward bend creates length and space in the spine. Many people have problems with some of these exercises. A good suggestion if you have problems touching the floor is to get a prop to help you reach down. As you continue in Yoga most people find that stretching this way, will eventually have their hands touching the floor without the aid of a prop in no time.

Backbends In Yoga:

Backbends in Yoga help open up the upper lungs lift the rib cage and many of these types of poses are supported by the abdomen. The spine also becomes more flexible and aids in body strength. There are many studies that show doing backbends actually help to stimulate the central nervous and immune systems along with realigning the spine.

These different types of poses help to shift energy which leaves the mind and emotions with more clarity and opens the heart chakra. Both backbends and forward bends are recommended for people who suffer from depression and anxiety.

How To Prepare For Yoga

Whether your yoga classes are at home or in a studio setting, there are basic dos' and don'ts we can go over in the way of preparation.

Studio Classes

- Check out some of the local yoga studios in your area and find out what type of classes they hold.

- Find out how long the teachers have been practicing.

- Ask to look over the studio and their facilities.

- Ask the studio if you have to bring your own props or does the studio supply them. By props we mean mat, straps or blocks.

- Ask what the studio requires from you in the way of etiquette and how long the classes run.

- Decide on a Yoga style that will work for you.

- Ask lots of questions because the teacher should know how to help you make the right decision.

- If this is your first time at the class let the teacher know, so he or she can keep an eye on your poses and help you to correct the alignment.

Beginners Props

If you are a beginner you will need a yoga mat, strap and maybe even your own block. A strap will help you with side leg lift poses and the block will help if you cannot yet touch the floor with forward bends. A block is a very effective prop for cobblers pose and extended stretches for the inside leg muscles. It allows for space between the feet and gives your inside thigh muscles more stretch.

Clothing

It really helps if your clothes can move with you. When you are in a forward bend a loose t-shirt will fall in front of your face making it hard to breathe properly, so you want your clothes to hug your body. There are plenty of suitable clothing styles which are sold for yoga and workouts. We are not telling you to wear spandex but be sensible about the clothing. Your legs will need room to freely move so you want to wear clothing that will not expose certain parts of your body. I am sure you get the point.

Hydration

If you are going to be doing a HOT (Bikram) yoga class you will need plenty of fluids. Average body temperature is 98.6° F or 37° C. The body naturally sweats when the core body temperature is raised. While there is a lot of humidity in these types of Yoga Classes, it actually doesn't help the natural sweating process.

Two hours before you attend a hot yoga class it is advised to drink at least 16 oz of water without any caffeine. During the class drink at least another 20 to 24 oz of water within the hour of the class. After the class is finished drink some more water. It is recommended that before attending any of these hot yoga classes that you are used to drinking 6 to 8 glasses of water a day on a regular basis to avoid any problems.

The hot yoga class will increase body fluid loss, so you really need to be aware of what you can physically tolerate. You do not want to have heat stroke or dehydration while in the class.

If you are attending a regular type of yoga class, it is still advisable to have a bottle of water on hand in the class for hydration purposes.

Eating

Do not eat a big meal before attending any yoga class. Only eat light foods and make sure there has been at least a two hour lapse before starting a class. Who needs to feel ill from a meal that has not digested correctly? When you are doing seated twists you will need the extra room for the abdominal area anyway.

An important point about bare feet

Spreading your toes out flat on the floor helps to balance your body better. This is an essential part of learning correct positioning in yoga. You will not be able to do this effectively if you keep sox and shoes on your feet.

Even if you are not attending a studio yoga class but have decided to do a home class with the help of a DVD, you will still need to make sure you have covered many of the same things we have just discussed in this chapter.

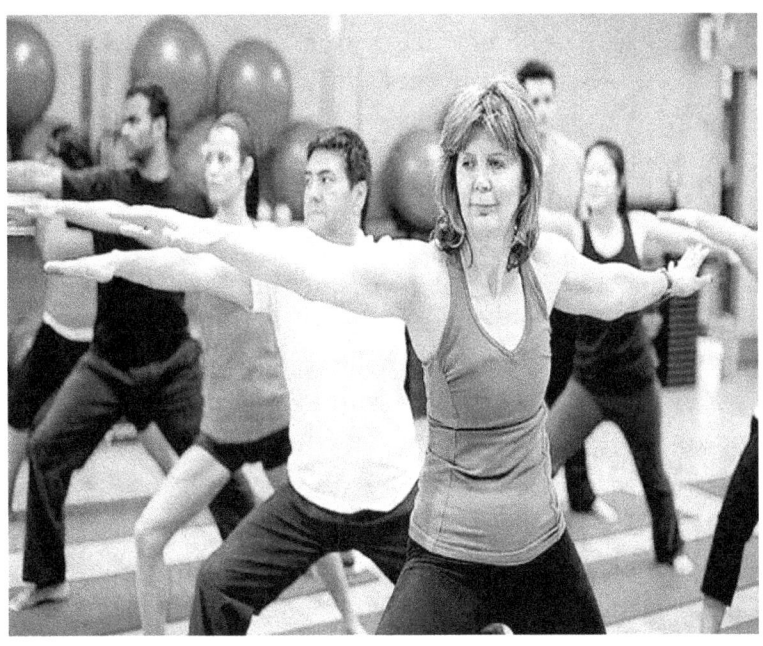

Beginning Your Workout

We cannot stress this enough for beginning a yoga workout; decide first what type of yoga you want to learn. Some DVD's for home practice will break up their asana into different categories. The student can then pick which class they want to apply into their practice for the day. We have already gone through some of the different types of yoga poses and what they do for the body.

What is your long term intended goals for Yoga? Is it to lose weight, gain strength, and have better flexibility or to have a better spiritual connection? Only you can answer these questions and you really should know each day what asana poses you will be practicing.

If you are tired you may want to use slower more relaxing movements. If you are feeling strong and healthy then challenge your body to more vigorous poses. Yoga is also about controlling your muscles, do they need strengthening?

Decide that you will practice a minimum of 3 days a week. Regardless of what movements you choose to use, Yoga is an expression of thought and feelings that come from within you. Therefore whatever asana (body position) you choose to use for the day it is because you have already decided this is the best choice.

There are plenty of great DVD's on the market that you can learn from. Make sure that you start off with the beginner's level and then work your way up. The exercises on DVD's are usually anywhere from 25 to 45 minutes in length. This is enough time for you to challenge your body and effectively learn your poses.

If you going to a studio yoga class, the positions will be varied and they will move from one set to the other. Most classes will last for about 45 minutes and there are usually a series of standing, seated, prone and supine poses, with a meditational cool down at the end of the class.

Poses And How To Do Them

We will take a few poses that a beginner and long time practitioner in Yoga can do. Many of these poses are quite popular to practice in a yoga class. They will work a wide range of muscles and help people with their strength and flexibility.

Sitting Forward Bend (Sukhasana)

This is a position even the beginner can do well. This is a good

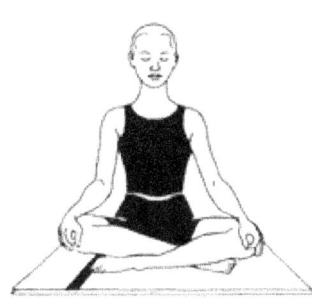

exercise for a restful sleep and should be practiced in the evening before retiring. The position reduces tension and opens up the hips and gives the body a sense of relaxation. If you have problems with your hips then use a pillow or rolled up towel to help position yourself better. If you feel one side of the body is uneven, use your hand to reposition the buttock and re-adjust your balance. Exhale and lean forward as far as you can with your arms in front of you. Do not constrict your breathing. Stay in the forward bend for a few seconds and release slowly back into an upright sitting position.

Standing Forward Bend (Uttanasana)

Stand with your feet approximately 6 inches apart, spread your toes into the ground and slowly bring your torso down to touch the floor. Do not push yourself and only reach as far as your body will allow. Take your opposite hand to the opposite sides of the elbows and stay in this position while bent. Relax and let your body just hang down. Sway from side to side just a little and

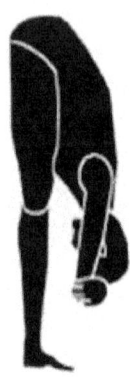

take slow deliberate

breaths emphasizing on releasing the breath slowly. You will find that the backs of your legs and hips will feel some relief too. This position can help people with sore shoulders, tension in the neck area and for people who have headaches and problems sleeping.

Down Dog (Adho Mukha Svanasana)

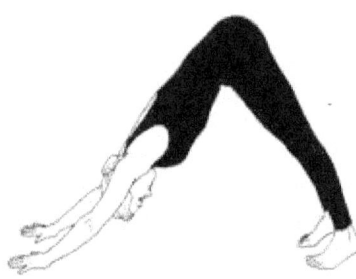

This is probably one of the most common yoga positions that you will get to know. Start on all fours in a hands and knee position. Bring your knees in line with your hips and your hands slightly ahead of your shoulders.

Exhale and slowly lift your knees away from the floor your legs only need to be hip width apart. If you can see your heals then adjust your position so that you can only see the toes. (It is not necessary to have your heals on the floor. You should feel a good stretch through your hips and the backs of your legs and calf muscles.) Lift your buttocks high and stretch while releasing your breath.

Your fingers should be spread apart and flat on the floor to balance the body better. You will feel the upper arms and shoulders helping to support your body weight as you stretch the legs back.

If you want to raise your seat higher, bend your knees re-position your feet again (Shifting slowly into position is good for the body. It helps to release tensions and aids in flexibility) and send the sitting bones high towards the sky. Now breathe slowly in through the nose and out slowly. Long intentional breathing is best.

Supine Butterfly Pose (Urdhva Shayana Patamgama)

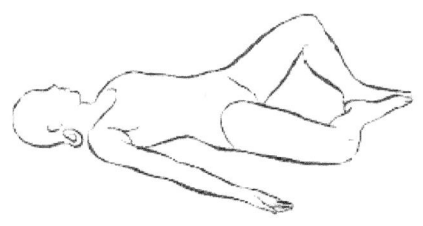

Lying on the floor bring your knees up with your feet planted firmly on the floor. Make sure that your chin is not higher than your forehead. Bring the soles of your feet together and slowly let your knees drift apart in opposite directions.

Inhale and slowly bring your knees back together, this pose should last 20 to 30 seconds before your knees meet together again.

Alternating Leg Lifts (Prthak Nalaka Udayama)

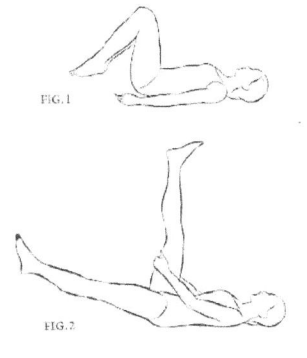

This pose will strengthen your abdominal muscles. Lie on your back with both legs extended on the floor. Again, make sure your chin is not higher than your forehead.

If at any time you feel any strain in your neck, place a pillow or rolled up towel under your head.

Bring both knees to your chest. Slightly hold your abdominal muscles and pull your navel in towards the spine. Keep the lower back in contact with the floor and do not arch it. Exhale slowly and lower your toes to the floor approximately ten inches from your bottom. Inhale slowly and bring your knees back up into your chest. Repeat this pose eight times swapping out opposite legs.

Mountain Pose (Tadasana)

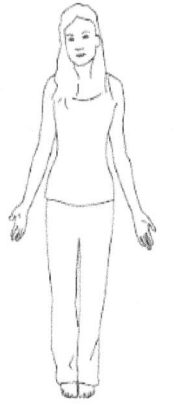

Stand with your feet hip width apart and big toes parallel to each other. Raise your kneecaps but do not lock or hyper-extend your knees. Keep your hands at your side ensuring that your arms are engaged and become as strong as your legs.

Lunge (Ardha Mandalasana)

Start this position in Mountain pose. Spread your toes into the ground, as you exhale and bend forward at the hip into a basic standing forward bend.

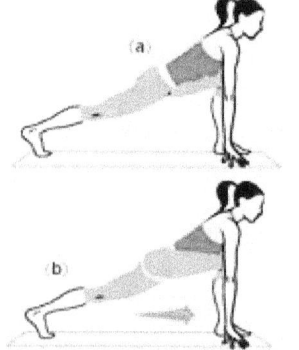

Place one leg back into the lunge position with only the front of the foot on the ground, while the heel remains extended in the back.

The knee of the front leg should be in alignment with your ankle. Place your hands shoulder width apart on either side of the front foot. You can either place your hands flat on the floor or to raise the body a little higher use your fingertips.

Drop your groin and hips evenly towards the floor. Stay in this pose for a few seconds, then release. To come back out of the pose you can either move the extended back leg forward to meet your hands, or move the bent leg back to meet the extended leg while placing your hands firmly on the ground. Swap your leg positions out and repeat the pose again.

Bridge Pose (Setu Bandha Sarvangasana)

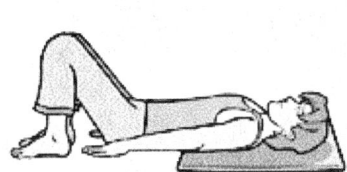

Lie down on your back with your knees bent and your feet hip width apart. Place your hands near your hips with the palms facing up.

Make sure that your feet are firmly pressed into the ground with toes spread apart.

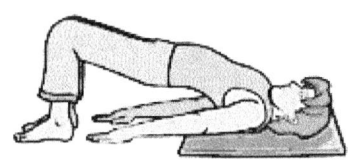

As you slowly breathe in, rise your torso up into a bridge position. If you can, reach your hands in underneath your body and clasp them together, while keeping the hands on the floor. Hold for approximately 5 seconds and then slowly release with your hands back to your sides. Drop your body back down onto the floor slowly and exhale as you release. Do this at least 3 times.

Stress Relief Relaxation Yoga

We have discussed in this book what great health benefits Yoga can have to people who suffer from depression, anxiety and stress. It is important to understand how to breathe correctly through some of the poses which will help to greatly reduce and even overcome these problems.

There are specific yoga poses which are designed to help relieve stress to the body and we have touched on a few. The forward bends, back bends and twists can greatly help to relieve stress. These poses bring a calming effect to the nervous system and help to bring tranquility the person. They relieve pressure in the spine and help to flood the body with much needed oxygen with the help of Ujjayi breathing.

Ujjayi Breathing

This is a breathing technique used in many different Yoga

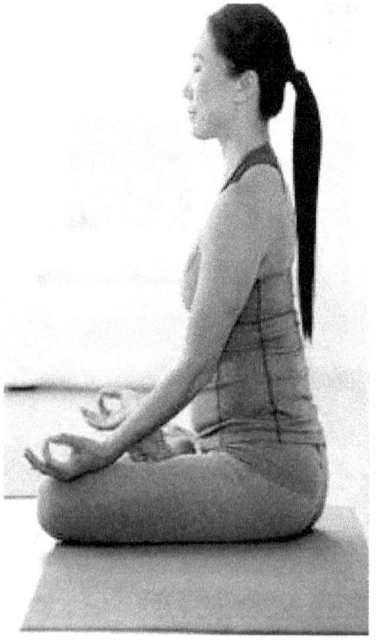

practices. Ujjayi is an intentional breath which helps with meditation and proper form with different yoga positions. It oxygenates the body and creates internal body heat. The Ujjayi breathing is also reported to regulate blood pressure within the body and can make a great difference to people's health.

The breathing technique actually slows your normal breathing to a more concentrated inhale and exhaling style. As a person breathes in and out they should hear a deliberate sound, almost as if there was a constriction in the windpipe.

This is the intentional slowing down of breath through the nose. The breath comes and goes from within the diaphragm, so the breathing can be controlled better. It's almost like sipping in air and then releasing it slowly from way down inside your body.

You may have heard Ujjayi being called the "the ocean breath". Ujjayi breathing is commonly used throughout Ashtanga, Vinyasa, Power Yoga and Flow Yoga.

Practice Makes Perfect With Breathing

In a seated crossed leg position, take one your hand to your throat (at the base of the throat) and the other to your diaphragm. Breathe in slowly almost feeling like your throat is constricted. There should be a sound that comes from the constriction.

Breathe in as far as you can and feel your diaphragm opening and expanding. Hold the breath for a couple of seconds and release slowly. Feel the breath being released from your diaphragm, back into your throat and through your nose. Again you want to hear the "ocean" sound as the air is being released.

Practice Ujjayi breathing a few minutes before starting your poses. This is the correct way to start your Yoga practice in calm and rhythmic way by using the Ujjayi breath.

Meditation Centering

For many people meditation is more important to practice during Yoga than the poses themselves. Meditation whether it is through prayer or peace from within the body, is crucial if one is to heal properly.

Because Yoga is more than just movement it does require dedication to understand the total body, mind and spirit. The chakras are constantly referred in yoga practice with the emphasis being on the heart chakra when the hands are placed in the prayer position.

Meditation can be done daily if one desires and does not always have to be attached to yoga. Visualization through meditation is very healing. If someone is suffering from depression and feels hopeless, meditation can be very soothing. Yoga has so many positive results with healing the mind.

We have a few suggestions which can help a person deal with problems and health issues. Turn off any harsh lights and use a candle, light some incense and even play soft, gentle music. If you wish to do this outside, find a calm place in nature away from distracting noise. These are calming and soothing things which can help with the energy flow around your body.

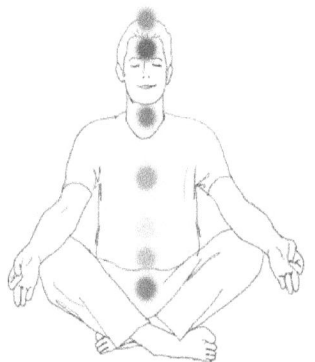

Sit in either a simple cross legged pose or lay down in corpse pose. Place your fingers in the "ohm" position resting on your knees. (See the graphic image) If lying down, place your hands in a comfortable position on the floor with the palms facing upward. Start by slowing your breathing down till you feel calm and relaxed.

Visualize healing light flooding your

body and concentrate on what ails you. Even if you are in good health you can still do this by simply flooding your body with healing energy. See the energy going around the body in great circles and touching all the chakra points in the body. Start with the base chakra and work your way up slowly.

Work within this type of meditation for about 10 minutes.

Meditation does not need to take a long time to be effective. 10 minutes every day should be all you need to center the body, control the emotions and feel more relaxed.

What happens with most people when they start practicing meditation is the feelings of inner peace are so wonderful that they want to do it again. Eventually when you feel ready, meditation can last longer and become more intense as you connect from a spiritual point of view.

Previously we touched on 2 forms of Yoga that incorporate the spiritual aspect. Kundalini and Kemetic Yoga can be practiced more as you increase your awareness through meditation.

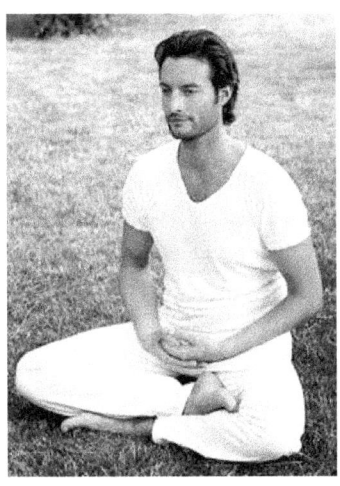

Conclusion

Through this book we have shown you how to proceed with a successful yoga practice. It is obvious that many different forms exist for people to choose how to best apply this amazing way of living into their lives.

Yoga is a conscious choice of poses and the end result is always to heal, strengthen and bring awareness into an individual's life. To call Yoga just exercise is to miss the greater awareness that centers on inner peace and bringing someone into their full potential.

You may have initially started Yoga to become more fit and that is a great start. We would encourage you to also think further into the healing and awareness aspect of all conscious thoughts and deeds. The true purpose of Yoga incorporates everything attached to mind, body and spirit into our daily lives.

We wish you all the best with your journey into Yoga and may you have many healthy years of inner peace, healing and happiness.

Namaste